Caregiver Book
A Simple Handbook for Caregivers

Jane John-Nwankwo RN, MSN

DEDICATION

Dedicated to all Caregivers

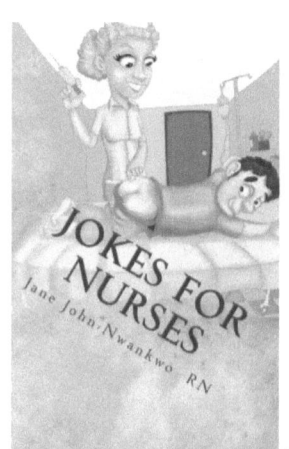

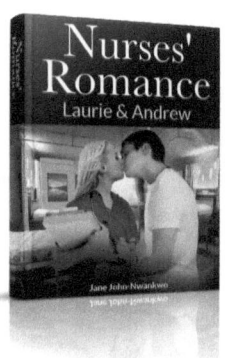

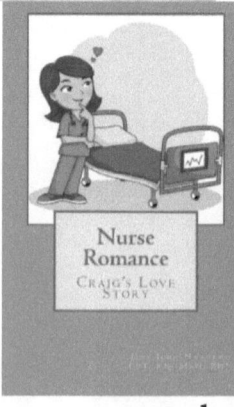

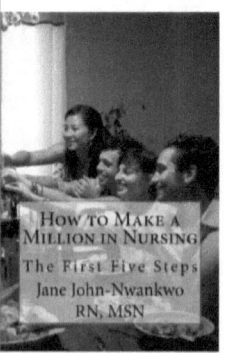

Have you purchased these books?

The Home Health Aide Textbook

Home Care Principles

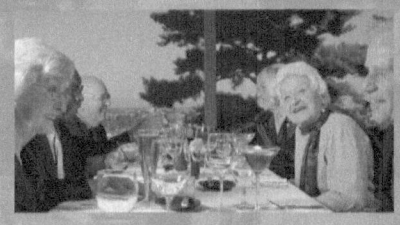

Jane John-Nwankwo
RN, MSN

Jane John-Nwankwo

HAVE YOU BOUGHT THESE BOOKS BY THE
SAME AUTHOR?

1. All the books in the 'Nurses' Romance' Series

2. All the books in the 'How to Make a Million in
    Nursing' Series

3. Director of Staff Development: The Nurse
    Educator

4. Crisis Prevention & Intervention in Healthcare

5. Work at Home Jobs for Nurses

6. Jokes for Nurses

7. All the books in 'Exam Prep' Series

Visit www.janejohn-nwankwo.com

PART ONE: The Ideal Caregiver

Who is the ideal caregiver?

The ideal caregiver is someone who fulfills all the following roles and qualities:

1. Knows his/her responsibilities
2. Knows his/her limitations
3. Carries out his/her job professionally
4. Maintains personal hygiene
5. Maintains punctuality
6. Maintains his/her own safety
7. Has good observation skills and good initiatives
8. Very open to suggestions
9. Has a sense of humor
10. Takes pride in his/her job

Responsibilities

The responsibilities of the caregiver include but are not limited to the following:

- Routine personal care
- Hygiene assistance
- Laundry
- Cleaning
- Shopping
- Meal planning and cooking
- Rides to doctor appointments and errands
- Medication reminders

Limitations

The caregiver should know that he/she is at this home to care. She/he is not biologically part of this family and as such does not have certain rights. There are times when she may have access to a patient's personal information like bank accounts, social security number, some Identification cards, and other private information. The limitations of her job must always come to his/her mind. These information should not be discussed outside the home of the patient. The information should not, in some cases even be discussed with the patient as he/she may become suspicious and start feeling uncomfortable around her and possibly dismiss her from the job. The caregiver is not to make certain decisions for her patients. When some vital decisions are to be made, the patient's son or daughter or significant other should be called to make the decision.

Professionalism

The free online dictionary defines professionalism as "the expertness characteristic of a professional person";" skillfulness by virtue of possessing special knowledge". [1] From this definition we can simply say that being professional means that one knows the skills of her jobs and delivers them with expertise. For a caregiver, do not feel intimated that you are serving, be very humble and carry out your responsibilities with expertise. The way you present yourself determines how you are valued and respected before your client. Remember that respect is not demanded but commanded. It is also very imperative that caregivers use appropriate clothing to work. Very tight fitting jeans or pants should be avoided. Revealing tops should also be avoided. The best clothes to wear to a caregiver job are scrubs.

---

[1] http://www.thefreedictionary.com/professionalism

I remember a certain day that a caregiver walked in and the aroma of the environment changed. I thought in my mind "Does it mean that this lady cannot perceive this odor?" I looked at the faces of those around me and I saw 'that look'. Other people were as uncomfortable as I was but no one dared told her what was happening. I started imagining what would happen when this lady bends over a patient to take care of him/her; that poor patient will definitely not find it funny! Should we maintain personal hygiene as caregivers? The answer is a bold YES! There is no such excuse as "I was late so I forgot to shower" or statements of that sort. Better be late and clean.

Punctuality

According to wordnetweb, punctuality means "the quality or habit of adhering to an appointed time"[2] Caregivers need to adhere to the appointed time for the start of shift. I once interviewed one of my

[2] http://wordnetweb.princeton.edu/perl/webwn?s=punctuality

clients, and the old woman commended a caregiver I sent to her "She is always her by 9 am, very punctual!" That made me feel very good as the employer. Sometimes caregivers could meet traffic or things of the sort. In order to maintain punctuality leave your house earlier than you should to give room for traffic emergencies. The issue at hand is your arrival on time, not the excuses that made you not to.

Maintenance of safety will be treated as a different topic.

Good observation skills and initiatives: Do you know the game 'bingo'? If you have played bingo or knows about it, you will remember that it requires a lot of alertness both in quick observation of the numbers and the ability to shout bingo first. The care giving job is a little like bingo because it demands a lot of observation and alertness. This patient has been left under your care. Erase it from your mind that she/he can stay without you; have it your mind that as far as you are in that house she is under your care and so deserves your complete attention. Observe for mood changes, signs of hunger, pain, etc. which she may feel uncomfortable to voice out. Ask open ended questions like "I see that your face is not very bright, is there something you want to talk about?" Be very polite and do not push for the patient to give you the information that she does not want to. Initiative means embarking on new ventures. In the case of senior care, I would explain it to mean the ability to think fast of the solution of an immediate problem. An example is this: you find your patient slump all of a sudden while eating at the dining table, what do you do? Many ideas run through your mind like "Run!" "Call the daughter or son" "Call 911" "Call your agency" "Start CPR". All these ideas are very vital and should all be done (except of course,"Run!") but should be placed in the correct order and this is the correct order: "Call 911", "Start CPR" but if you suspect a fracture, stop and don't move the patient. When the emergency team arrives, call the significant other then call your agency. In the case of an emergency as described, be sure to give accurate information to the emergency team. Give as much correct information as you know and only those needed for the care.

Openness to suggestions

The caregiver must be open to suggestions given by her agency and the family. It is always good to remember that you are there to serve.

Has a sense of humor

When I started practicing as a nurse, I would come to work, take my duties so seriously, trying to be the best nurse, do my job and go home. As time went on, I started finding out that my colleagues were not very comfortable with me. Why? I soon found out: I was 'too serious' with my work. It was not until I brought my real funny self and started expressing my sense of humor that everyone started changing their minds about me. There is more to life. Season every second as much as you can. That will make you enjoy your job and feel at home to leave your house the next day. Moreover, that will make your clients want you to always be there for them.

Takes pride in the job

Have you ever seen someone who hates his job? He makes a lot of mistakes at the job, creates a lot of bad impressions, gets depressed on the job and never retains one job for too long. I want to say that the care giving job is a noble profession because it is not everyone that possesses the gift to care for others. So, my dear caregiver, take pride in your job!

"The caregiver needs to feel good about themselves. If you don't feel good, you won't respond well to a difficult situation."

Kathleen O'Brien

<u>More explanations on the ideal caregiver</u>

A caregiver can be anybody who helps a person when he/she is in need of it. In general, people suffering from acute illnesses need the help of caregivers. An ideal care giver is one who in addition to looking after the patients, also helps them with their grocery shopping, house cleaning, cooking, shopping, paying bills, giving medicine, bathing, using the toilet, dressing and eating. Individuals who do not charge a penny when it comes to take care of patients are referred to as family caregivers or informal caregivers.

If your loved one is suffering from any acute illness, you can be by his/her side to help. Most health centers may need patients to have a caregiver for helping them throughout the treatment. As a caregiver you need to provide emotional support to the patient. In addition to this, you need to also act as his/her advocate. As a caregiver, your prime responsibility lies in playing a viable role in the treatment and recovery of your loved one. You need to learn more about your patient's /patients' disease as well as treatment options as it will help you to make good choices about your care.

Role of an ideal care giver

As a caregiver, you need to remember that you are an eminent member of the heath care group. You need to play a viable role all through the patient's treatment starting from planning to recovery process.

It is quite obvious on your part to feel thrown into a strange world of test results, treatment choices and medical terms if your loved one is suffering from any acute disease. You may have to gather all possible information on earth about the disease, consult doctors, and stay by your patient's side supporting him/her. In simple words, that's what we call an ideal caregiver.

Each patient's needs are different. For example, a patient suffering from autism will have different needs when compared with a patient suffering from Alzheimer's disease. Hence, as a caregiver you need to find your own way of catering to those needs. Irrespective of the different needs, at the end of the day what is expected from an ideal caregiver is love and support throughout the treatment, recovering or peaceful death procedure.

Taking up the responsibility of being a caregiver may turn out to be an overwhelming job. In fact, it helps if you are aware of your job and responsibilities.

- As a caregiver, your first job involves finding out the expectations of the hospital or rather the doctors from you. Many health centers provide special sessions for helping caregivers learn what they need to do when it comes to taking care of patients. For home caregivers, you need to find out the expectations of the family from you.

- Talk to your patient about what they need. For instance, some patients may need only emotional support from you and leave the task of talking to doctors as your advocate to others. On the flip side, some patients may ask you to take up their complete responsibility starting from grocery shopping, giving medicines to providing emotional aid.

You need to act as your patient's advocate. In other words, you need to act as an active supporter of your patient. You can act as your patient's advocate in a number of spheres such as:

- Medical: Being an active member of the health care group, your job lies in gathering information, talking to the physicians together with taking care of the patient at the time of his/her recovery.
- Financial: If your patient has asked you look after his/her financial matters as well then you may talk to insurer and manage health costs as well as routine household finances.
- Emotional as well as social: Be by your patient's side and listen to what he/she has to say to you.

You can maintain regular updates about your patients in any way that can only be accessible to you. You can write down the names, maps, phone numbers, questions, instructions, and much in a diary. As a caregiver, you need to see to it that medical team answers all your queries. If you can't be available when the doctor pays a visit to your patient, you can fix a time according to your convenience for talking about your patient's progress to the doctor. Don't be scared of asking questions regarding the patient's progress till you get a satisfactory answer. There are quite a few things that may take place just as expected. Complications may take place and the recovery period may last for quite a long time than expected. You may come across situation when you need to re-admit your patient no sooner you have brought him/her home. An ideal care giver is one who plans for setbacks, surprises as well as delays. Try focusing on things that you may manage at present and measure the progress of your patient in small increments.

There is a lot to care giving even after the patient leaves the clinic or hospital. In fact, the real care giving job starts off at this juncture. During the first weeks or months after your patient returns home, things may not be that normal. Being a caregiver, you job involves administering medications, Changing colostomy bags, checking the patient's blood sugar, as well as monitoring the patient for infection as well as other complications. Taking the care of a patient at home is much more challenging as compared to taking the care of a patient when at hospital.

Family members as well as friends may not always understand the hard core truth that difficulties never come to an end after the return of the patient from the hospital. In fact, this is the time when a patient needs maximum support from the care giver.

While dealing with a patient, your prime responsibility lies in maintaining an optimistic outlook and a good sense of humor. It is true that dealing with a patient suffering from acute illness is not a matter of joke, but many caregivers know that by maintaining a good sense of humor, they have helped patients to cope up with their illness.

An ideal care giver adjusts to the needs of the patient

The need of a patient at the time of the diagnosis will certainly differ from his/her need at the time of the recovery procedure. An ideal care giver is one who is familiar with the changing responsibilities well in advance. Over and above, this approach of his will help in carrying out the below mentioned transitions more conveniently:

- Helping your patient in preparing for the treatment

- Care giving at the hospital

- Care giving after the patient returns home

Sharing your care giving responsibilities with others

For caregivers who are part of the family, you may

try sharing your care giving role with others. Even if you play the chief role in managing the aforementioned areas, you can always delegate some tasks to others. In fact, if you want to be an ideal caregiver, then you need to take utmost care of your own self as well. Hence, it would be advisable on your part if you assign small tasks to others and use your energy in helping the patient which they need you the most.

Often, an individual acts as the main caregiver of the patient. Despite this fact, at times it becomes difficult to carry out the task single-handedly. To avoid this situation, a group of individuals can work jointly as caregivers. When a group shares the role of care giving, communication and organization are keys to success.

Meeting your own needs as care giver

Many a time, caregivers neglect themselves while taking care of others. This could work out for short-term care giving but in long term care giving, It definitely will lead to problems. Some problems that could occur when caregivers put themselves last include but are not limited to: 1. Their becoming ill, 2. Their hating the job 3. Their becoming depressed. 4. Their not delivering appropriate care to their care recipient and thus suffer both themselves and the care recipients.

One of the problems that caregivers usually face is the problem of time. When someone starts the job of care giving, it will not take long to discover that the extra time that was once available is no longer there. This is a big issue and that is why the solution needs to be discussed. Have you ever wondered why the united states made 3 12-hour shifts the full time job for healthcare professional (for those who run 12-hour shifts)? This is because they want to prevent the burn-out associated with care giving. I cannot count the number of times that I forgot to eat while I was working in the hospital. It will start by my saying "I will eat in 15 minutes" and then 15 minutes turns to 30 and 30 turns to 2 hours and sometimes no food till the end of the shift. I cannot count the number of times I had to run into the pantry just to grab an apple juice because I my body needed some food. I did not do this every day but I certainly cannot count how many times I have put myself last. From my inquiries, this is not just MY PROBLEM, it is the problem of many caregivers – putting ourselves last.

 In order to prevent the burn-out, frustration and depression that accompanies care giving, it is vital to keep some time during the day for yourself. When I learnt this principle, I would gladly hand over my responsibility to the next person and go for lunch or just for a break. In home care, it will depend on the number of hours required of you, if you are doing a four to six hour job, then you can do without a break. But if it is longer, find time to take care of yourself. I remember a day in the hospital that two nurses were quarrelling because one nurse was almost urinating on her herself while the other was still in the restroom. The question now arose "Why did this nurse wait till the last minute before going to the restroom to urinate" The answer is simple. She put herself last. In home care, find time to go to the restroom when it is safe so that you do not endanger the safety of the one receiving your care. Imagine holding a patient in your hands who is depending on you not to fall and at the same time, you are trying to hold back your Urine from dripping on your pants!

Meeting your own requirements is important as well. In other words, if you want to be an ideal caregiver, then you need to stay in good health.

An ideal caregiver is one who in addition to taking care of the patients, takes care of him/her as well.

When a person is diagnosed with an acute illness and is struggling in between life and death, people are so engrossed with the patient that they often overlook that most important partner of the patient, i.e. the caregiver.

Caring for a person suffering from an acute illness often turns out to be an emotionally draining as well as physically challenging venture. Watching your loved one passing through strenuous medical procedures may change the mind of the most optimistic and healthiest caregiver. Not only this, some care givers feel that their physical health has declined to a considerable extent over the years due to the physical and emotional strains involved in the care giving job. To avoid these consequences, this book introduces some vital points that would help them in meeting personal needs as care giver.

- Care giving is a responsibility and breaks are your deserved right. Hence be sure to reward your own self with occasional breaks.

- Look out for symptoms of depression and never delay when it comes to seeking professional help. The sooner you got better, the sooner you will be able to take care of your patients.

- If people come forward to share your responsibility as a caregiver, don't hesitate. Instead assign them simple tasks that they can carry out easily. You can assign them some of the daily as well as weekly tasks.

- Talk to your friends or try spending some moments away from the patient. You can utilize this time in doing anything that helps you feel relaxed. Check out something that reminds you about the most pleasurable moments of your life.

- Talk to someone who can provide you emotional support. Friends and family members are of great help at this point of time. They are good listeners with whom you may share your feelings. Professional counseling, talks with support groups and clergy are also good ways of support.

- Concentrate on the significant tasks, keep your energy reserved for helping your patients with things they need the most.

- You can't be an ideal caregiver if you are sick or exhausted. Hence, try eating well balanced meals, exercise regularly and sleep well. Devote some time for your own self. Whether you go for a movie, a walk or visit your friend place, your prime objective should be to take out some time for yourself.

- Ask your family member or friend to act as your advocate, in the like manner as you act as your patient's advocate. Your advocate may keep an eye on you and provide you with the support as well as the time you crave for.

- Appreciate your own self for your care giving job. At times, people are so busy with the patient that they simply turn a deaf ear towards the effort put forward by the caregiver. At times, even the patient is too tired and sick to reward your efforts.

- Take adequate care of your back as your care giving job may demand too much of pulling, pushing and lifting.

- Have faith in your instincts as they are most likely to show you the right direction.

It has been mentioned earlier that individuals who do not charge a penny when it comes to take care of patients are referred to as family caregivers or informal caregivers. Let us now check out a couple of suggestions to help family caregivers when it comes to taking care of the patients.

- As a caregiver, you need to jot down all your queries in pen and paper so that you don't forget them

- Try being clear when it comes to talking about the patient to the doctor. Don't ramble up things at this juncture

- If there are innumerable queries that you need to discuss, they try going for a consultation appointment. This approach allows you as well as the physician to discuss the progress of the patient in an unhurried manner

- Keep your own self updated about the disability or disease of the patient. You can also surf the internet for this purpose.

- Check out the routine at the hospital or doctor's chamber so that you can find a suitable time to discuss about the patient's progress.

- Keep aloof your anger and your sense of helplessness about no being able to help your patient.

- Keep in mind that the doctor will try his level best to recover your patient.

Care givers generally share a close if not too close relationship with their patients. Each caregiver and patient is in no way similar to each other. Over and above, the viewpoint of a patient is likely to differ from the viewpoint of a care giver. Hence, it would be advisable on your part if you try talking to your patient and in the process find out what he/she needs at each and every phase of illness.

An ideal care giver is one who adapts his or her service for addressing the needs of the patient. The patient and the caregiver need to discuss their expectations (i.e. what sort of responsibilities they need from each other). If possible, they can also jot down their agreement in pen and paper in the form of an agreement. For being an ideal care giver, you need to know the difference between doing and caring. Welcome ideas as well as technologies that promote the independence of your patient. Try updating your own self about the condition of your patient and make sure to communicate with the doctor in an efficient manner.

Good communication is believed to be the most viable quality of a caregiver. In fact, this quality turns out to be more important when caregiver is an immediate family member. There may be times when the patient feels hesitant to speak about his/her actual health condition simply because he/she feels that by doing so he/she will burden the care giver.

An ideal caregiver is one who is an expert in time management skills. Often they need to cope up with full time jobs in order to take care of their loved ones. In addition to this, they need to also monitor the financial stress that goes hand in hand with care giving. It is true that the life of a caregiver is full of challenges, but there are innumerable rewards as well. In fact, in the care giving process, most caregivers develop a better relationship with the patient they are looking after. Moreover, adequate care giving makes an individual spiritually as well as religiously sound. In a nutshell, care giving leads to stronger relationships and helps in maintaining an optimistic outlook on life. The difficulties that come with care giving may be overcome with effective communication.

The rewards that come with care giving often make up for the hardships associated with it.

Keeping Yourself Safe As A Caregiver

The following areas should always be borne in mind by the caregiver for safety:

1. The five senses

2. Information

3. Sexual behaviors

The sense of hearing: Sound is an important alert for safety. It can indicate that your patient has fallen, that someone is trying to break into the house, things of the sort. The caregiver must always be sound alert. When left alone with your client and the doorbell rings, do not open the door if you do not know the person. Some bad person may know that everyone has gone to work and you are left alone with this sick person, and so decides to trick you into opening the door yourself which, of course will not trigger alarms.

The sense of sight: This has earlier on been mentioned under observation skills. Careful observation should part of the caregiver's skills. Some examples where the sense of sight could be tools for safety include the observation of unusual movement around the house which could be a criminal, observation of your client to see changes in his mood and behavior on time, take the necessary actions, and save yourself troubles that could arise out of your neglect.

The sense of touch: Always react to any feel of undue wetness. If this is noted on the floor, dry it without waste of time to avoid falls, if it is on the bed, or diaper, change the client to avoid pressure ulcers. Using your sense of touch, always take note of your clients temperature becoming warmer than usual. Could he or she be having a fever?

The sense of smell: This tells you if something is burning which of course should be investigated shut off to avoid fire. It may also tell you when your patient is wet.

The sense of taste: This will be mostly used if you are preparing meals for the client.

Information: Keep watch for useful information that could affect both your safety and the safety of the caregiver. This could be information on fire around the neighborhood, flood, earthquakes, and the sort. Any information that could hamper your safety or that of your client should be of paramount importance to you.

Sexual Behaviors: Bear it in mind that a lot of caregivers have had issues of sexual assaults in their records and that many of these people are probably innocent. So, in order to keep yourself safe during the care giving job, avoid comments or behaviors that can easily be misunderstood. An example is when changing the diaper of an old man, and you observe his penis, forget your professionalism and start asking him if he was circumcised. Also avoid touches that may be misunderstood as sexual harassment.

More information on keeping yourself safe as a caregiver

Caregivers' minds encircle with questions but with the call of their duty, they forget to distinguish that there are some things which are beyond their limit; they try to achieve them and unfortunately in the process they tend to lose spirit and motivation and thus their mental and physical health deteriorate. Caring for an individual who is suffering from a severe disease can be challenging. Specially in case of caring for Alzheimer's disease or any related dementia, there is the possibility that the caregiver can become frustrated and irritated. If they are ignored and not treated, they can become apart of every caregiver's life and that ultimately can lead to serious consequences for the person the caregivers care for. Thus, it is not only necessary for the person the caregiver is caring for but it is also important for the self- belief and the satisfaction of a caregiver's job.

Why care for a caregiver?

Frustration often arises when a caregiver tries to change some uncontrollable situations and this frustration can even arise from any daily activities like bathing, dressing and eating. When a caregiver is taking care of some serious cases like the bone marrow or cord blood transplant, it can be really stressful. The patient's behavior can also become irritating to caregivers. Examples are when a patient is wandering or repeatedly asking questions, the caregiver has to be patient and overcome their frustration and stress because at the fact is that the caregivers are entrusted with the duty of caring for the patient and not the other way round. If you are a caregiver, taking care of yourself is not only about taking out 15 minutes and spending some time with your friends. Rather it is more about finding someone, who will be able to give you an emotional support and can really motivate you to get your fit into the role.

A Caregiver's Life

The caregiver's stress can lead to an emotional and physical strain, thus leading to frustration and anger while taking care of the patient. In some cases, the person may feel guilty thinking that he/she is not able to deliver the best of the care to the patient. There may be feelings of loneliness and exhaustion. These mentioned factors can lead to serious complications, but the good news is that these complications can be avoided.

The warning signs

Some of the signs of frustration are:

- headache
- chest pains
- lack of patience
- stomach cramps
- knot in the throat
- compulsive eating
- shortness of breath
- increased smoking
- desire to strike out
- regular alcohol consumption

For combating all these symptoms it is necessary that a caregiver should respond to an extreme frustration and for doing that, you need the following:

- help yourself to learn the signs and the symptoms
- intervene or calm down physically
- thought modification process can be helpful for reducing your stress
- assertive communication is necessary
- seek help

When you are caring for others, the precautionary steps are different for different diseases. There are even some precautionary steps which you should take for yourself. So make the process easy. It is necessary that you should make some plans that will help both you and the care recipient.

Keeping yourself safe

Caring for yourself should be your first love because when you are able to love and care for yourself then you can assume the role of a caregiver. Thus watching for the warning signs for the frustration is important as you can intervene with the immediate activity to calm down. Claming down is necessary when there are any tensed situations involving the patient. Trying out these simple processes could be helpful:

- Count one to ten slowly and take few breaths
- Take a brief walk to another room and collect your thoughts
- Any uncontrollable situations should be left for the moment and if possible avoid any self reaction
- You can even try reading, praying, meditating, singing, music or taking a bath
- Practicing relaxing techniques at last for 10 minutes in a day

If possible, try to recall the whole situation and replay in your mind al that happened and what you should have done to make the situation better.

This is a very useful too which will help to reduce some of the stress from the job. There are many situations which affect how you feel and there can be feelings of frustration from any such difficult circumstances. If you are able to analyze these situations, and follow the thought patterns which are adaptive in nature then there could be a build up of self defense against frustration. Also trying to transform unhealthful thought patterns into adaptive and positive thought patterns can also be useful. Some of the common thought patterns are:

You can tend to take up some negative thoughts and multiply it with something else, for example when you are becoming ready to take the patient to the doctor, the car breaks down and you tend to think that something always goes wrong whenever you are taking him/her outside.

You tend to overlook good situations and hardly ever think about motivation like "I can do more", rather you capitalize on the bad moments.

Sometimes you may even jump to a conclusion without being aware of the facts. You tend to think of others thinking negatively of you and your duties and thus you unconsciously show that in your actions.

As said earlier, take pride in your job, motivate yourself and make the most of the moment. Carry out your duties in such a way that the client will see you as the "ideal caregiver".

One of the most important things for the caregiver is to have the right amount of sleep because deprivation of sleep can cause moodiness and thus it might affect the care giving process for the patient. Quality sleep is important and it is not just about the hours you sleep, it is more about the requirement of the body. Since care giving job may involve getting up early in the morning and remaining alert throughout the day, perhaps you need more sleep. In many cases, the caregiving duties are split into shifts like night and day shift.

When you are not on 'duty' make sure to take enough rest. If it happens that you are the only one that does all the shifts, ask for help, so as to rest yourself and be healthy to meet the demands of the job.

Some of the common ways of decreasing your stress as a caregiver could be explained in a nutshell, like the following:

1. Arrange a meeting with your family when a loved one is diagnosed. This will enable each family member to decide on how much they can contribute towards a paid caregiver. That way, you will not suffer because you are the only one at home with the senior.

2. Self-care is necessary because if the caregiver becomes ill, the entire care giving process is disrupted. If the caregiver is not well, then it is better to handover the task

to someone else who's trustworthy, someone from the family or from outside.

3. It is necessary to take care of the stress levels which you are facing in the process of caring for the patient. There could be some early warning signs for potential problem and it is important to check them out so as to maintain the care giving process.

4. Meeting physical needs: When you are taking care of someone, it is important for you to be 100% fit and sound and this can be possible when you are consuming proper healthy food, having sufficient rest and have time for recreation and relaxation.

5. Honesty counts: If you feel that you are not being able to meet the mental and physical demands of the care of the patient, being honest with your inabilities will certainly help you.

6. Making legal and financial plans on the forefront. It is necessary to take care of the

advance directories like Health Care Surrogate, Living Will and Power of Attorney will help you to take care of the business in advance.

7. Realistic approach: Be hopeful but keep yourself grounded with the realities of the moment. It will help you to reduce your stress up to certain level when you are able to balance the hopefulness and realities relayed to the condition of the patient.

8. 100% Not possible: it is wise to accept the fact, that there can be certain situations where you may not be able to provide 100% percent to your loved one or one who is the patient. Be cautious and never overdo anything because that might cause problems to the patient and thereby enhancing your stress level.

9. Avoid guilty feeling unnecessarily: Learning to say NO is not a guilt and there could even be times when you won't hear the word

THANK YOU, however, be patient and learn to deal with feelings of grief and anger.

10. Praise yourself: you are not a super hero or a saint, but as a human being you have given your best and you have been able to handle numerous responsibilities with great deal of stress. So, praise yourself even if no one else does.

Communication skills

Good communication with the patient or to someone related with the patient is very important. It helps you to know what is expected of you and makes you feel safe to express yourself so that others could understand your limits and needs. The process of Assertive Communication is different from Passive Communication or Aggressive communication.

"Passive communication is a form of expression that is ineffective and maladaptive. Those with a passive communication style are generally afraid of confrontation and do not feel they have the right to make their wishes and desires known. This style of communication can lead to feelings of anxiety, anger, depression and helplessness and is common among those with social anxiety disorder (SAD)."[3]

"Passive communication is based on compliance and hopes to avoid confrontation at all costs. In this mode we don't talk much, question even less, and actually do very little. We just don't want to rock the boat. Passives have learned that it is safer not to react and better to disappear than to stand up and be noticed."[4] From the descriptions given about passive communication, it is clear that this is not the type of communication that the care giver needs.

[3] http://socialanxietydisorder.about.com/od/glossaryp/g/passive.htm

[4] http://www.angelfire.com/az2/webenglish/commstyles.html

"Aggressive communication always involves manipulation. We may attempt to make people do what we want by inducing guilt (hurt) or by using intimidation and control tactics (anger). Covert or overt, we simply want our needs met - and right now! Although there are a few arenas where aggressive behavior is called for (i.e., sports or war), it will never work in a relationship. Ironically, the more aggressive sports rely heavily on team members and rational coaching strategies. Even war might be avoided if we could learn to be more assertive and negotiate to solve our problems"[5]

Having seen the above two types of communication, we may want to look at assertive communication. "The most effective and healthiest form of communication is the assertive style. It's how we naturally express ourselves when our self-esteem is

intact, giving us the confidence to communicate
http://www.angelfire.com/az2/webenglish/commstyles.html

without games and manipulation. When we are being assertive, we work hard to create mutually satisfying solutions. We communicate our needs clearly and forthrightly. We care about the relationship and strive for a win/win situation. We know our limits and refuse to be pushed beyond them just because someone else wants or needs something from us. Surprisingly, assertive is the style most people use least."[6]

Some of the important keys to assertive communications are:

- Respect your own feelings, desires and needs

- Speak about your feelings without any hesitation, shame or humiliation

- Use 'I' statements rather than 'You' statements

[6] ibid

- Use words like "Its important to..." rather than using "should" in your statements

When you feel that that it will not be possible for you to continue as a caregiver, then it is better to accept this fact because that will not be favorable to you alone but to the patient as well. It is wise to discuss your needs along with the family members and friends and you will be able to share the care giving responsibility. It is quite natural that people will not realize when you need help or assistance. Therefore you should take the initiative to ask for help and express your needs. If someone offers you help don't refuse because there could be errands or task when you need to attend to.

More information on communication

When your loved one is suffering from diseases like Alzheimer or Dementia, it can be really an uphill task to get the right communication. It is usually

very difficult to convey the message across their
senses and if they are not able to perceive, that
you cannot blame them for because the decreased
level of perception is consistent with these types of
patients. There can however, be certain times of
the days which can be worse or better; when they
will be able to understand what you want to
communicate and respond accordingly. There can
be also be times when they sit still and it will be
like talking to a stone idol. Whatever may be the
case it is necessary to understand their needs and
demand, understand them and communicate
effectively. So here are 5 positive communication
techniques which will help to get your message
right across towards the patient and thereby can
fulfill the caregiver's duty towards the patient.

- The first and foremost thing that is
  necessary is to put ourselves in their shoes.
  Yes, that is essential because unless you are
  able to understand their problems and
  inabilities, you won't be able to take off the
  righteous methods to communicate with
  them. The person suffering from dementia
  needs to be knowledgeable about his/her
  disease and that should not be done by
  force. Rather there is no need to give them

any "gentle reminder" or "correction" because that could be psychologically damaging. It is better to congratulate them rather than correcting them as it will be easier to cope up with the situation. So improve this part of communication with them and offer them with the support and validation they want.

- Another important factor which you need to keep in mind is to place the right kind of communication with the health care providers. It is necessary to convey all the problems and difficulties the patient faces. Recognize and demonstrate wellness habits of the patient to the doctor. You need to recognize all the signs and symptoms of the common chronic illness and have to abide the process of treatment and the lifestyle changes that is required for the managing the chronic illness.

- Using effective communication techniques and strategies for the older adults and recognizing and responding to the challenging behaviors of the older patients. If you are not well aware of the communication techniques, you can plan a doctor's visit and learn communication practical skills from them to conduct an effective communication with the doctors, nurses, home health workers and health care providers.

- Allow the elder person to express their feelings because it will help them to disclose some hidden feelings of significant loss. If they don't express they will tend to develop sadness and grief and may in turn lead to more deterioration of their health. Sit with them and try to make a space so that they don't hesitate to share their inner feelings.

- Since an elder patient has various life experiences, it is important for them to allow the person with thoughts and it is necessary to listen and respect them.

Try out these techniques as they may be challenging at times but it's worth the effort.

Cultural Sensitivity in Home Care giving

Performing a routine task for the toddlers or

patients is similar to what we generally do for our own family. The point is to be at the demarcation line where care giver services are to be peddled but keeping the professionalism intact. Caregivers need to be aware of cultural differences that why I have chosen to address it in this book. Conflicts should be avoided because of cultural differences, that is why the caregiver should do an "assessment" of the client at the beginning of her job to know what the client likes and what she/he does not; to know what he believes in or does not. This will encourage a smoother communication and help build a therapeutic relationship faster. Listening carefully and respectfully to the values and beliefs of the patients and respecting them in your day to day activity is what is referred to as cultural sensitivity.

Culture is referred to as "the way of life of the people". I knew this definition from my high school so I do not know the source. So, when we are saying that the caregiver should be culturally sensitive, we are saying that the caregiver should respect the way of life of her client! Culture is made of values, beliefs and practices and they are shared by some group, children inherit culture from their elder ones and it lasts throughout adulthood.

Advantages of cultural sensitivity

- Person becomes competent and confident
- A stronger connection with the client and the family members.
- Families share a trusting relationship with the caregiver.
- Effective meeting with families and children
- Expansion of knowledge
- Avoidance of conflicts

Follow these simple tips and avoid conflicts with the patient:

- Reflect on the care giving practices and analyze the things which are being done or performed
- Observe the interactions of the close ones and relatives with the patient
- Differences may arise with the relatives but it is better to acknowledge them as it will reduce anxiety and confusion.
- Ask for more information and learn about the relatives and close one's perspective and clarify every point of view. This will help to handle situations or any issue arising from the patient's abnormal behaviors arising out of cultural sensitivity.

Communication is the best way to negotiate with any differences arising out of cultural sensitivity. So check out these few tips:

- Build a trusting relationship with the close ones and relatives of the patient
- Determine the level of commitment necessary to resolve the problem
- Identify problems in words and decide the plan the action

Escorting and Transporting Your Patient

Dealing with patients requires a lot of care and professional expertise. Escorting and transporting a patient implies monitoring the mental and physical state of the person during the whole journey. A person who is escorting and transporting a patient is fully responsible for observing any signs of discomfort or anxiety during the journey. In the event of any kind of discomfort or anxiety the care giver should take all the required steps to alleviate the cause of discomfort with the help of their skills and expertise.

Escorting a patient should not be confused with accompanying a patient to a destination. Both tasks are different from one another and they should not be confused. A person's relative or friend may accompany a person whereas escorting a patient is a professional role and hence this task is generally conducted by professional care givers like health or social care professionals.

Before transporting a patient the personnel who is handling the patient should make sure that the client is properly dressed for the occasion. If the destination is the doctor's office or the mall, it is important to dress the senior with a cardigan to guard against the coldness usually associated with these areas because of the air conditioner. While in the car, make sure all buckles and button have been pressed. If the person is on a wheel chair, makes sure the knots holding the wheelchair to the floor of the transport has been knotted. If it is a car, make sure the seat belt has been put on. Whatever the case, your security, as well as the security of the client are of paramount importance.

Before escorting the patient the care giver should be familiar with the appropriate destination well in advance. The anticipated time of return should also be discussed with the patient and in the case of delays the mobile and phone numbers of the concerned people or units should be with him or her.

Escorting and transporting a person are generally for the purposes of attending an appointment e.g. to a doctor's chamber, court or housing department, requiring an assessment outside the hospital for e.g. home, transferring from one place to another or taking the patient to an inpatient department of a medical unit.

A person who is escorting and transporting a patient should be aware of the medical history and the clinical condition of the patient. There should be provision for water as while traveling the patient's mouth may become dry. Toilet and food breaks should be ensured in consultation with the patient throughout the journey. Medication should be provided as prescribed and if the medication should be taken with food there should be a stop for food during the journey.

After the escort and on return the care giver must make an entry in the patient's record. The record should contain elaborate details identifying the reason for the escort, the patient's behavior and the outcome of the escort. The details of any accidents or incidents that occurred during the escort should also be recorded in the patient's records. In home care giving, if there were no incidences, there will be no need to make any records.

The above mentioned points should be taken into consideration when escorting and transporting a patient. They require a lot of care and attention and more importantly the understanding and love of the care giver who is taking care of them.

Fire And Safety Preparedness

Every year there are innumerable residential fires that lead to damage of property or loss of life. Well damage to property can be recovered but what if someone loses his or life. As an ideal caregiver your prime responsibility lies in adapting fire and safety measures and protecting the client in case a fire breaks out. By adhering to a fire and safety measures and being vigilant a homecare giver can lower the risk of a fire break out to a considerable extent.

Some of the probable reasons of a fire break out are smoking, cooking, and a couple of other fire hazards. Let us now take a closer look at how an ideal home care giver can prevent fire break outs from taking place.

Cooking

- While answering a phone call or stepping out of the house the burner should be turned off
- While handling hot pans and pots oven mitts should be used
- While preparing a meal, the cooking oil should be heated in low flame
- Avoid putting flammable towels as well as mitts on the stove

Smoking

- The lighter and old matches should be disposed
- The matches, cigars as well as cigarettes should be kept at a safe place
- Make sure the patient never lies down while smoking or consuming alcohol

- Dropped butts needs to be disposed in large tin cans at the earliest
- For the elimination of ashes, large ashtrays should be used

Additional precautions:

- Ask a professional to clean the fireplace chimney frequently
- Opt for extension cords that come with circuit breakers. Avoid overloading the circuit breaker
- The electrical cords should not hang from the book shelves
- The electrical panel should be inspected on a routine basis. You can appoint an expert electrician for this purpose.
- A good quality security system needs to be set up in your house
- The yard as well as the house should be well lighted
- If you are escorting the patient to the hospital, make sure there is someone to keep an eye on the house
- The yard, garage as well as home needs to be free of rubbish as well as combustible items
- There needs to be a provision for a fire extinguisher in the house
- The windows as well as the doors needs to be free from obstructions for easy and safe exit

- A smoke detector needs to be installed in the house
- The electric smoke alarms should be checked on a consistent basis
- Try cleaning the alarms after every six months
- The battery of the alarms needs to be charged at least once in a year
- Close the doors and windows closed while the patient is asleep as this provides some prevention against fire

It is hoped that the aforementioned suggestions will help an ideal home care giver in preventing his/her patient as well as other members of the family from the disasters caused due to a fire break out.

Phone Etiquette As A Home Caregiver

Telephone is a part of daily activity and for a caregiver, it is part of the requirements of the job. Since it is a part of the areas where caregivers have to walk and talk, there are certain things which are essential to follow as a part of the telephone etiquette. In every good care giving course, telephone etiquette is a part of the curriculums. This is because this particular etiquette is certainly important to prevent treating the elderly or the people on the other line rudely or abruptly while using the modes of communications. This helps in conveying any emergency problems to the doctor or to the family members. In the process, there can be the possibility of the caregiver showing bad manners while speaking on the telephone to address the patient's problem. That is why good etiquette is needed.

There are can also be tendency to be too short or become 'the salesperson' in most of the telephone calls. Have you ever had an experience with someone who just rude on the phone? Or someone that wants you to explain things hundred times up to the amount of frustration? If you have had any of these experiences, then you will understand why the caregiver needs to adopt good phone manners. Politeness and simplicity is not the only manners needed in conducting proper phone etiquette, there are certain other things as well.

Talking of the proper way to answer the telephone, except "hello" nothing is accepted as the proper way to start addressing the other person on the phone when answering from ones house. Using words like "Yes" is considered inappropriate in telephone etiquette. The individual calling tend to draw quick conclusion and therefore the person sounds cold and aloof and will hesitate to communicate effectively. So as a caregiver, when you are calling some person it is better to address them properly and generally it is better to start this way: "May I speak to Mr._____ please," and in case the person who is being asked for is not present in the house then a proper way to tell "I am sorry Mr._____ is not available at this time, Can I take a message?" Don't utter anything abrupt like "NO" because that reflects your negativity on the caller. Even if someone calls the number of your client mistakenly, it is better not to hang up, but to politely say "I am sorry, but this is a wrong number."

When you are making a telephone call to the doctor or to the relatives of the patient at odd times like late in the night (Any call after 8:30 pm is considered late), it is necessary to be patient and courteous while describing the person's emergency. In case of wrong dialing of the number, expressing apology is a must. When you are not with the patient, and you are communicating him/her on the telephone, it is important to be patient and calm with your voice to get across the message to your patient.

In a nutshell, here are few of the Phone etiquette tips as a home caregiver.

- Be very calm, calculated and patient on the phone
- Remember that you are representing your client, so be very professional
- Do not pass out your bad emotions to persons on the other line
- Dialing wrong numbers demand prompt apology and not hanging up abruptly
- Calling any business nearing the closing time should be avoided if possible
- When you are calling any health professionals or doctor, keep your calls short and informative as they are generally busy people

PART TWO: Common cases found in home care giving and how to deal with them.

Ten ways to prevent falls for seniors in the home

Do you know that nearly fifty percent of the falls experienced by seniors take place in the home itself? Well, there isn't any need to get worried as I have some good news for you: all you need to do is bring about a couple of improvements and modifications in the senior's home. Also following the suggestions included here will help to prevent your seniors for innumerable common hazards that may lead to disabling or in rare cases fatal falls. These suggestions are sure to help seniors lead a safe life.

With aging, the risk for falling increases because their senses dim and nervous systems tends to deteriorate. Elderly people often suffer from weakened vision and the balance mechanism in their ears becomes less accurate. The sedentary lifestyle of theirs may lead to muscle loss, thereby leading to falls. In seniors, even a minor fall may at times lead to fractured bones.

Now without beating about the bush, let us divert our attention on how to make our home a safe to live in place for seniors:

- Bathroom...a risk prone place! That's true...falls are more commonly to take place in bathrooms...hence it would be advisable on your part to set up bath benches in your bathroom so that seniors are at a lower risk to slip. Also arrange for toilet risers, toilet safety frames, grab bars and tub and shower treads. Well, I guess you get me...I intend to say that you need to make your bathroom slip resistant. How? Well, that's a good question, I must say! To begin with, for adding steady support in case of slippery situations, you need to install non-slip strips on the shower floor or tub. In addition to this, you need to place non-skid mats on the floors of your bathroom. You can also look for garb bars that have been approved by the ADA.

- Falls among seniors can also be a result of dim light or poor vision, particularly in areas such as basements and stairways. So how can you avoid that? Well, your first step lies in installing brighter light bulbs throughout your house. It would be better, if you opt for bulbs with greater longevity as they'll never burn out at a time you need them the most. Opt for bright lights for your bedrooms, bathrooms, stairwells and hallways. While new fluorescent bulbs have a greater longevity as compared to the conventional incandescents, yet despite this fact some may not like the light that they deliver.

- Go for motion-sensor switches which turn on lights automatically while entering an area. You can also go for light switches which glow; hence you can look for them easily during the dark.

- Make sure you install nightlights close to the floor for lowering the chances of falling or tripping while you need to pay a visit to the bathroom during the nighttime.

- Another way through which you can help seniors from tripping is by clearing off the debris from hallways, stairs and walkways.

- Try removing the scatter rugs. If you fail to do so, then it would be ideal on your part to secure the rags to the floor using heavy duty and double-sided tape. You don't have to wander hither and thither in search of these, simply walk up to any hardware store and order for one!

- You can play safe with the stairways if you paint a white strip (ensure the measurement is somewhere around two inch) on the top of the each step's edge. Try using a gritty paint as it helps your seniors in staying more surefooted while they move up as well as down. This isn't all...seniors are at a greater risk to fall from the carpeted steps as well. But you can avoid this problem if you use white colored non-skid tape.

- Keep an eye on the electrical cords and make sure they don't obstruct any foot paths. Don't overcrowd the cabinets, bookcases and shelves. And make sure they aren't too high. This approach will prevent the seniors from using a stepladder or stool while taking off things from the cabinets, bookcases and shelves. Try placing a chair or bench close to the entrances as this will provide you a secure and handy place for setting down bags, or sitting down while slipping your shoes on as well as off.

- Get their vision and hearing checked on a routine basis. In other words, start the check ups even before noticing problems. Consult with the doctor about the drug therapy for ensuring that after taking it you won't feel dizzy.

- Elderly people should avoid standing up quickly as this may make you feel dizzy and probably fall. Prior to standing, try wiggling your feet and toes and swing your legs, if needed. Try exercising on a routine basis as this helps in strengthening your muscles as well as improving your agility. However, prior to this make sure you consult your doctor.

- Before standing up, try moving enough so that your blood pressure and heart rate increases. And last but not the least elderly people should limit their consumption of alcohol.

With aging, the risk for falling goes on increasing. It is true that most of the falls lead to minor injuries, but at the same time nearly ten to fifty percent lead to fractures as well as other serious injuries. Falls may take place anywhere, but a senor may more commonly experience it in the home. To be more specific, falls are likely to take place while getting out or climbing the bathtub.

In addition to elderly people, people suffering from weakness in legs or feet, problems with balance and walking, arthritis, particularly in the knee, problems with vision or hearing, dementia, low blood pressure, dehydration also run at a greater risk of developing falls. In a nutshell, the more risk factor a person is prone to, the more are their chances of falls.

References:

http://www.facebook.com/note.php?note_id=102231026244&ref=mf

http://www.allegromedical.com/blog/prevent-falls-at-home-with-home-safety-products-955.html

http://brighamandwomens.staywellsolutionsonline.com/RelatedItems/1,820

Prevention of falls for Seniors (contd)

Falls are one of the common occurrences in a person's life as they grow older. There are many reasons that can cause a fall for seniors. It is indeed a big problem and falls can sometime prove to be life threatening. There are many people who are affected badly by the falls resulting into permanent injuries. Injuries that can result out of falls are broken bones, head injuries and even accidents that harm the interior body parts. Head injuries can be more damaging than any other falls and can cause problems like memory loss or blood clot.

Falls for the seniors can be easily prevented if we use some of the prevention tips that help to cut down the accidents. Let's look at some of these valuable tips:

a) Enroll the seniors for an exercise program: Now, body fitness is a big thing when it comes to preventing falls. Seniors can enroll for fitness programs that would make them physically fit thus reducing the chances of a fall. One can on the yoga or Tai Chi classes as they are neither very taxing on the body nor provide very tough regimens to follow. Fat and unfit bodies are more prone to falls and the only way to avoid these is regular exercise. Exercise can also help to reduce fat and provide the necessary fitness to legs and hands. It is better to practice the yoga moves or exercises that help to improve the strength of the leg muscles. You can seek the help of an expert or doctor in order to guide you choose the right exercise program.

b) Safe home to live at: Falls at home is a common thing and most of the falls occur at or homes. You must remove the objects that can cause you or the seniors at home to trip. Things like books, shoes and other objects can cause real problems for the seniors as there is a fear of tripping over them. Use tapes to stop the rugs from slipping over. Try to put the daily use items in the closet and keep them at a height that you or the seniors can reach easily. Install the grab bars beside the toilet or bath tub. The mats that one uses should not be slippery and try to wear the shoes that are not slippery and provide a good holding on the ground.

c) Get an eye check: You need to ensure that the seniors have a proper vision and the only way to so is to get it checked by the doctor. The doctor can provide glasses or lenses that would improve the vision if there are any such problems. It often happens that seniors keep on wearing the same glasses for long without getting their eyes checked. Now this is a sure way of getting falls. Proper and regular eye checkup is necessary for the aging eyes.

d) Get your medicines checked: You need to get the medicines of seniors checked by the doctor as they may be taking medicines that make them drowsy. You need to be a little more careful about the medicines to avoid the falls for seniors.

The care of a person in the early stages of Alzheimer's disease

Alzheimer's is a common form of dementia in which a person faces problem with their memory or thought process. Memory or thought related problems can affect anyone irrespective of their age or sex and when this starts hampering daily life activities then this can mean real trouble. The changes can even affect the personality or the mood of the patient. The number of dementia related cases is somewhere near 4 million and out of this 2/3rd suffers from the problem of Alzheimer's disease.

It is often seen that we forget about an incident that might have occurred only a few moments back but this is not the soul symptom of being affected with something as serious as Alzheimer's. The former case may be a simple problem of a temporary memory failure where the brain fails to recollect information. The symptoms of Alzheimer's are divided into two broad categories: Early stage and late stage. In the early stage, the patient faces the frequent loss in memory (mostly the ones that are related to the recent events and conversations). We even get to see problems like repeating questions, problem with speaking a language, writing and even using a few objects. Depression and changes in the personality can also occur and there are also problems with spatial orientation while walking or driving. These problems keep on increasing with time and take an acute shape and this is what forms the symptoms for the later stage where people face almost complete memory loss. For instance, they forget why they have come to a particular place or why they are walking etc.

There are no straight treatments available for the problem of Alzheimer's and only proper care can make the lives of the patient's easier. It is really a challenging task to take care of a patient with Alzheimer's disease and this can at times prove to be tougher than one can think. A caregiver would face new problems everyday and they have to adapt themselves to the fast changing demands of the patient. The behavior pattern of the patient changes and the caregiver needs to make a lot of changes in their caretaking procedure to get acquainted to the new set of demands. Here, we are going to look at the things that can make your job of taking care of a person in the early stages of Alzheimer's a little easy.

After your family member or loved one is detected with Alzheimer's, you need to start making changes in your lifestyle and the place you reside, so as to make things easier for the person. Changes are necessary in order to create an environment where the patient would be physically safe and at the same time would feel comfortable. You need to restructure the social lives of the person as it won't remain normal with every passing day. The environment of the home needs to change so as one needs to understand that things won't remain the same anymore. The ways of communication also needs to change and development of new ways of communication should be emphasized upon. For instance, one needs to have prior scheduling for visits to the patient in order to avoid surprise, but this doesn't mean that one needs to snap all social contacts with the Alzheimer's patient. One also needs to make a proper structure of the daily activities that are to be performed by the daily living. One also needs to help out the patient make social contact on a regular basis. You need to set up a safe environment in the home so that the patient does not meet with any accidents at home.

The condition of the patient deteriorates as the days pass and one should understand that the patient becomes emotionally fragile. The emotional support needs to come from the side of the caregiver and this can create a sense of well being in the patient. Even emotional support help to allay the fears and anxiety that build up in the mind of the people who suffer from Alzheimer's. It is better not to use logic in order to alleviate the fear in these patients as they lose their capacity of rational thinking. The risks of accidents and injuries would increase with time, so it is better to be always prepared for them. It is better to rearrange the house to avoid any types of untowardly incidences.

You need to be sensitive towards the patient as there are going to problems that can make your job tougher. If you want to inform the patient about the diagnosis then it is better to do that in a roundabout manner. Do not directly tell the patient that they suffer from the problem of Alzheimer's and instead tell them that it has something to do with their memory problem or anything better that comes to your mind. You should be patient enough while dealing with the queries of the patient and if you are performing a task that the patient is supposed to perform then try to explain to them why you are doing it.

You need to have a positive attitude towards seeing improvement in the patient and should not get bogged down by the initial setbacks. Patients who are in the early stage of Alzheimer's would get worse as they move to the late stages, so one should be ready to expect worse things. If you are taking care of an Alzheimer's patient then you need to communicate with the patient in a way that they can rely and have faith on you. Be supportive to the patient not only when they show up the negative traits but also appreciate if he does anything new or good. You need to understand that these patients are going to have behavioral problem but you also need to be ready to cope up with the same.

Taking care of the Alzheimer's patients is certainly not an easy task and one needs to take good care of oneself in order to provide the best support to the patients.

The Care Of a Person in the Late Stages of Alzheimer's Disease

Alzheimer's and its late stages require a complete different approach in the care of the patient. The care does not get restricted to providing emotional support and taking care of the simple needs but it now shifts to a more complex environment. You need to take round the clock care of the patient and there is hardly any room for leaving the patient alone. In the later stages of the disease, it progresses in a disorderly fashion and this is why there is a need to take care of the patient in a proper way. This time is very crucial for the caregivers or the people who take carte of their Alzheimer inflicted loved ones. It is very challenging to take care of the patients who are in the late stages of Alzheimer's disease. It is often seen that a caregiver gets so attached with performing their daily duties but this is the time when they need to accept the bitter reality that death is a reality that is not very far away from their loved ones. The sense of bereavement can at times make the caregiver mentally weak but they have to gather themselves in order to perform their duties properly till the last breath of their loved one.

One should understand that despite the best care and treatment their loved ones are slowly nearing death.

The late stage of Alzheimer attacks the patient so badly that they are not even in a position to communicate properly and they are completely dependent on the caregiver. They are bedridden and look forward to their caregivers even for their daily requirements. This is the time when they lose all their memory and do not remember even their loved ones with whom they might have spent happy days even a few years back. They become more and more dependent on their caregivers as they are not even in a position to verbally let their needs or requirements known.

You must know the fact that at the late stage the patient of Alzheimer's is not at all in a position to sit, talk, walk or eat and they even cannot make any sense of the world around them. This is the time when the caregivers go through a testing time. They have to take care of daily activities of the patient like bathing, feeding, toileting and dressing. You have to be in a position to take complete care of the patients and this is the time when the caregivers also need to be mentally as well as physically fit.

Memory loss in the Alzheimer's disease doesn't mean that the patient loses their feelings. They experience normal feelings like fear, sadness, peace, lonely, loved etc. Now, you are the only person who can provide solace to the patient and you are also the one who can allay all their fears and discomfort. It is best to not leave the patient alone while they are awake as they would not be able to communicate their feelings but their bodily gestures may provide you with some hints.

In the late stage one can even look at the other options for patient care as it is not always possible to keep the patient at home. Looking at the physical safety needs of the patient or the need for an advanced treatment, one has to find a hospital or care center where the patient can be under 24 hour monitoring. The decision to keep a last stage patient at home means that the caregiver has to have a lot of mental strength and complete family support without which there is no way a person can stand the jitters. If you are keeping your loved one at home then you need to make a world of changes in the way you have been living and also the place where your loved one lives. The patient's needs for the changes are to be first jotted down so that you do everything to make the adjustment of the patient pretty easy. It has been often seen that the people who are in the early stage do not face problems with adjustments, but patients in the late stage can feel completely lost with minor changes. Well this is attributed to the fact that the late stage patients do not have the ability to remember even the smallest changes around them.

Here are a few things that would help you to understand whether you are in any position to take care of an Alzheimer's patient:

a) See if you are in a position to take a 24 hour care of the patient or not. This is very important as you need to understand that Alzheimer's patients in their last stages require complete support even for their smallest daily activities.

b) Find out whether your room has the provision for a hospital bed, Commode or wheel chair.

This is because the patient needs to move as less as possible.

c) Is there a proper transportation support so that the patient can be moved whenever any emergency crops up?

d) You also need to judge whether you possess the necessary stamina to lift or carry your loved one or not.

The last stage of Alzheimer's completely cripples a person both mentally as well as physically, so you have to mentally prepare yourself to be close to a person who cannot even communicate his daily needs in a proper way. There is a bit difference in reading about the difficulties and actually experiencing the same from close quarters. The care giver has to be very attentive to catch even the smallest gestures of the patient to understand their requirements. One has to be so habituated with the patient that there is not even a single movement of the patient that misses one's eyes. One needs to learn some soothing techniques like massage, fragrance, music and touch so as to provide a holistic comfort system to the system. The people who perform the job of a caretaker should themselves have a support system as they are the ones who have to witness the agonizing days of the patient before they finally expire. If you are a caregiver then you must learn to get proper grip over your emotions and become mentally strong.

Autism And How To Care For An Autistic Patient

We have very often come across the term "Autism" in our daily lives. There are many of us who have heard the term however we are still not sure about what it actually implies. In general autism is a persuasive developmental disorder that impairs a child's normal development of language, communication and social interaction skills. Many are still unaware of the actual causes of the disorder and its treatment options. The subject of autism has been one of constant research and there have been many scientific breakthroughs in its diagnosis and treatment process.

Autism is a brain disorder that deals with an abnormal self-absorption with oneself. It is marked with communication disorders and a short attention span. Autism involves restricted and repetitive behavior in patients and the signs of autism begin when a child is three years. There are two other autism related disorders which in medical terms are called Asperger Syndrome and Pervasive Developmental Disorder - Not Otherwise Specified (PDD-NOS). Both of these disorders fall under the category of Autism Spectrum Disorders or ASD.

- Asperger Syndrome: The patient displays significant difficulties in social interaction coupled with a series of restricted and repetitive behavioral patterns. Those afflicted with autism are physically clumsy and they frequently use a typical form of language.

- Pervasive Developmental Disorder - Not Otherwise Specified (PDD-NOS): PDD-NOS is a milder autism disorder. In this disorder the patient does not suffer from all the symptoms of autism.

Autism and both the Autism Spectrum Diseases are complicated neurodevelopment disorders and its causes are still not definitely proven. A lot of research is still on and medically doctors are of the opinion that autism is a genetic disorder. There are some rare cases where autism is caused by some birth defect causing agents. There are some that are of the opinion that certain after effects of vaccines may be the cause of autism however such hypotheses have no scientific evidence and have not been convincingly proven.

One can easily identify the early symptoms of autism in children. Autistic children display comprehension and language development impairments. They respond poorly to name and they have deficient non verbal communication for example they lack appropriate emotional gestures, ignore people, prefer to be alone, lack of pointing and problems with following a point, lack of social interaction skills with others etc. The indicators of autistic behavior in very young children are no babble, pointing or gestures by the 12th month, no single word by the 18th month, no two word spontaneous phrase by the 24th month and any loss of language or social skill at any age. Autistic children either ignore or have a very friendly attitude with adults. They tend to prefer loneliness and they love being in their own imaginary world. They prefer solitary activities and they have a social imagination that they generally do not share with others. They have social impairments and they are over sensitive to moods and touch. They tend to play repetitive games with toys, for example lining up of objects and the turning on and off of light switches despite repeated scolding.

Autism can also be present in adults and normally the Asperger Syndrome disorder sometimes transits into adulthood too. This type of autism is called classic autism and there are many people who are unaware of these traits in adults. Autistic adults function independently and on most occasions also obtain college degrees. Psychiatrists and pediatricians in the past and sometimes even today are reluctant to pronounce adults as autistic out of compassion for their parents. These adults have poor living skills and are either reclusive or eccentric. They have a level of social awkwardness and they tend to prefer being on their own. They may be unable to care for themselves and fail to comprehend the social behavior of others. They are generally obsessed with a particular subject and they tend to bring the topic of any discussion back to their interests. They tend to become angry if they cannot do what they want or if they are stuck in a schedule that disinterests them. They are generally not empathetic and do not understand the emotions of others except their own. People with autism also have problems with keeping the track of time when they are engaged in activities that they like doing the most. They tend to stack and organize things on shelves and they love to do solitary activities. Autistic adults have a lack of emotional control and though their emotional outbursts may not be like a child it can be very irritating to any normal person or bystander.

One cannot physically identify a person with autistic traits however when communicating with a patient one may be able to ascertain the levels of autism as its levels differ from individual to individual. Some physical characteristic of autism may include:

- The face has low muscle tone
- The eyes may be large with pupil dilation
- The skin is pale
- The tendency of banging one's head
- The tendency of slapping one's ears
- The motor skills of the patient are impaired.

Children with autistic tendencies have problems painting, coloring, solving jigsaw puzzles and doing other normal classroom activities like normal children. They are very slow in development than other normal children. These characteristics may differ from one child to another and in most cases therapy can make a difference to treatment in these patients. The following are some important real facts about autism that are beneficial to understand the disorder more clearly:

- Autism occurs in one of every 150 births
- After cerebral palsy and mental retardation it is the third most common developmental disability in the world.
- It occurs more often than the diseases of childhood cancer, cystic fibrosis, and multiple sclerosis.
- The disorder begins before the age of three years.
- Experimental regimens of diet coupled with mineral and vitamin supplements are successful as therapy and treatments are done through medical interventions and behavioral therapy.
- In many cases insurance companies do not cover or recognize various treatments for autism

- Significant improvements have been observed with the recent treatment and medical therapies.
- Both autistic children and adults live a normal life span

Autism is a spectrum disorder and the care of autistic patients differ from individual to individuals. There are no laboratory tests to confirm autism and one can identify its symptoms through a detailed developmental case history of the child and clinical examination. A psychological evaluation should be carried out by a professional to confirm whether a person is autistic or not. The psychologist generally conducts a series of autism screening tests to determine whether a patient is autistic or not. There is no hard and fast rule that autistic patients need to be treated with medicines. There are many effective strategies that can help one with dealing with these patients.

One should keep a notebook or a detailed journal about the patient. One should always track the developmental history of the patient. One may be asked to keep a set of questionnaires which will ask about the behavior and development of the patient.

Writing the daily developments of the patient will help one successfully keep track of the patient. Moreover one can also observe what can work and what cannot work with the patient. This notebook and journal comes in handy when the patient may be difficult to handle at times. It helps to identify the patterns for difficult times and the triggers for the problems that may be faced by the patient.

One should have a positive attitude when dealing with an autistic patient. There may be some days when the patient responds positively to therapy and on some days there may be reverse reactions. One should not be de motivated and discouraged with the results. One should be patient and have a very understanding attitude towards the autistic child or person. In the process one can also find out what thinks work for the patient and what does not. It helps in the long run as the person becomes aware of what he needs to avoid.

The autistic patient may have fixations like making repeated noises, staring at turning wheels etc. There may be some obsessions with objects, TV programs, animals etc. Control and tolerance of this behavior within controlled parameters can be a powerful tool that can help in the patient's educational, emotional and social instruction. One can relate to the interests of the patient and thus gain the confidence of the patient. This leads to acceptance of new things especially in children who suffer from autistic disorders. Using this time with the patient can help one relate and hence connect with the patient on a higher level.

When caring for an autistic child or patient one can find support in the company of other autistic caretakers and hence get essential help. There are many trusted individuals who can provide childcare and advice on how to deal with patients having the same disorder.

One can check with one State Health Department to check there are special health departments that can take care of patients with similar health care needs. One can also resort to visual stimuli. Most autistic children are visually oriented and very often they love to communicate with the use of sign language and pointing out to pictures in a special book that may be put together to help them communicate. Even an autistic child who speaks may be able to communicate better with the help of visual stimulus. If one wants to teach the child something the use of a picture book comes in handy and the child responds well to the technique. Some autistic children can repeat verbal instructions word to word however they are not able to convert their thoughts into actions. Pictures very often can help them to that and hence it is a successful mechanism for teaching autistic children. Autistic individuals often have poor auditory processing skills. As a result of this they often do not understand what people are saying to them. They tend to hear the words but they do not understand what the words actually mean. Very often the person's lack of understanding can lead to confusion and utter frustration to others. Very often this may also escalate into behavioral problems. Picture visual aids can also help them to a considerable extent.

Sometimes an autistic child may demonstrate behavior problems at school but not at home, or vice versa. For example, the parent may have already developed a strategy to tackle and stop such behavior at home, but the teacher is unaware of this strategy and the child continues to be troublesome. In such cases the parent and the teacher should interact on a regular basis to solve this problem in the child. If the child's behavior is bad at school but not at home there are many possible reasons for this behavior such as a lack of consistency. There are can be physical causes and it has been observed that cleaning solvents and florescent classroom lighting can trigger negative responses in autistic children. The janitors very often use powerful chemicals to clean classrooms and the smell of these chemicals remains in the class even on the next day. Chemical residues often induce negative reactions in very sensitive people. Children place their hands on chairs and tables and end up inhaling the smell. They may even wind up in the child's mouth thus making him sensitive. The chemicals affect the brain functioning and in turn behavior. It has been observed that after parents and teachers wipe the students' desks with water or a natural cleaning solution prior to class each morning, they have reported rather remarkable improvements in the behavior of autistic children.

One can check if there are any early intervention programs that are available in the locality. The school district authorities can be contacted for evaluation of the child and thus the child can be enrolled for any special pre school program on the advice of a specialist. Make can also make a special request to the local school authorities and check whether they have any special programs for autistic children. The child needs to qualify for the special program and one should make sure that the school has set up an individual Education Plan for the child. This document is a very serious document that ensures that the child gets the special service and education needs. The free and appropriate education that is given to the child is called FAPE.

One can refer to some good parenting theory books that will help in the treatment of autistic children. There are many guides that are available and one may take recourse to them for help.

Autistic patients both young and old need constant care and attention. Autistic adults can be classified into two categories and they are High Functioning Autistics and Low Functioning Autistics (LFA). There are numerous health care professionals and organizations that can offer valuable advice on how to deal with these patients.

The high functioning autistic adults are very successful and they live relatively normal lives.

They can work, care and support themselves and live independently with a family of their own. To lead a normal life the HFA adult must have had a proper education while growing up and if he has been effectively taught he can understand social behavior and responses. By the time the child reaches adulthood then he can adjust and contribute to society. Some high functioning autistics may still face or have to struggle with social interaction. There are organizations which health care providers that can help them and they can be consulted for support and guidance. The Low Functioning Autistics (LFA) need constant care and attention like autistic children. They too should be taken to health care specialists for guidance and proper progress evaluation.

There are a number of approaches that are used in the treatment and therapy of autistic patients. Some of the most popular ones are the structured and language therapy, social skills therapy and occupational therapy. Health care professionals' resorts to these natural therapy tools to treat patients and in the event of extreme cases they resort to medications. The healthcare professionals keep a daily track of neuropsychological reports to monitor progress and developments.

Autism is not a disorder to be dreaded and with professional guidance and personal evaluation a patient can lead a normal life. With family love and support an autistic patient can be successfully treated. Autism is not a disease it is a disorder that requires compassion, constant care and a supportive and understanding attitude towards the patient. There are many organizations that extend support and generate awareness on autism. Families of autistic patients can take recourse to these organizations and get invaluable advice and support for dealing with autistic patients and their well-being. Both parents and professionals can benefit from these programs and hence make autistic patients live a more better and fulfilled life.

REVIEW QUESTIONS

The ideal caregiver is someone who knows his/her responsibilities, maintain punctuality very open to suggestions and takes pride in his/her job

       A. True

       B. False

       C. Neither

1. The responsibilities of the caregiver include all of the following except

    A. Routine personal care hygiene assistance

    B. Prescribing medications

    C. Rides to doctor appointments and errands

2. _____ is define as skillfulness by virtue a possessing special knowledge

   A. Limitations

   B. Identification

   C. Professionalism

3. A caregiver should always wear tight fitting jeans or pants to work

   A. True

   B. False

   C. Neither

4. Should you maintain personal hygiene as a caregiver

   A. Sometimes

   B. Always

   C. Never

5. _____ means the quality or habit of adhering to an appointed time

A. Responsibility

B. Professional

C. Punctuality

6. If you find your patient slump all of a sudden while eating at the dining table what should you do?

   A. Call 911, start CPR, call your agency

   B. Run

   C. Just ignore your patient because you are just there to make money

7. An ideal caregiver does not adjust to the needs of the patient

   A. True

   B. False

   C. Neither

8. Some problems that could occur when caregivers put themselves last include all of the following except

   A. Meeting their own needs

   B. They become ill and hate their job

   C. They do not deliver appropriate care to their patient

9. The United States made three 12 hour shifts full time to burn out caregivers

   A. True

   B. False

   C. Neither

10. If you want to be an ideal care giver then you need to stay in good health

    A. True

    B. False

    C. Neither

11. As a caregiver you should keep your own self updates about the disability or disease of the patient

    A. True

    B. False

    C. Neither

12. Bad communication is believed to be the most viable quality of a caregiver

    A. True

    B. False

    C. Neither

13. The 3 areas involve in keeping yourself safe as a caregiver involve all of the following except

    A. The five senses

    B. Information, sexual behaviors

    C. Interrogating the patient

14. Some of the signs of frustration are

    A. Feeling happy

    B. Singing all the time

    C. Headache, knot in throat, desire to strike

    out

15. Calming down is necessary when there are

    any tensed situations involving the patient

    A. True

    B. False

    C. Neither

16. Any uncontrollable situations should be

    dealt with right away

    A. True

    B. False

    C. Neither

17. Some common ways of decreasing your

    stress involves all of the following except

A. Meeting physical needs

B. Praise your self

C. Going on a romantic date with your patient

18. Bad communication with the patient or to someone related with the patient is not important

A. True

B. False

C. Neither

19. _____ communication is a form of expressing that is ineffective and maladaptive

A. Passive communication

B. Aggressive communication

C. Good communication

20. The most effective and healthiest form of communication is the _____ style

    A. Aggressive

    B. Passive

    C. Assertive

21. Assertive style of communication is the style people use most

    A. True

    B. False

    C. Neither

22. There are ____ communication technique which can help get your message across towards the patient

    A. 3

    B. 5

    C. 7

23. The first and foremost thing is to put our selves in their shoes

    A. True

    B. False

    C. Neither

24. Listening carefully and respectfully to the values and beliefs of the patients and respecting them in your day to day activity is what is referred to as

    A. Cultural activity

    B. Assessment sensitivity

    C. Cultural sensitivity

25. _____ is referred to as the way of life of the people

    A. Norms

    B. Culture

    C. Beliefs

26. Advantages of cultural sensitivity involves all of the following except

    A. Avoidance of conflicts

    B. A stronger connection with the client and the family members

    C. Respecting your own feelings, desires and needs

27. Communication is not the best way to negotiate with any differences arising out of cultural sensitivity

    A. True

    B. False

    C. Neither

28. Escorting a patient should not be confused with accompanying a patient to a destination

    A. True

B. False

C. Neither

29. A person who is escorting and transporting a patient should not be aware of the medical history and the clinical condition of the patient

    A. True

    B. False

    C. Neither

30. Some of the probable reasons of a fire breakout are smoking, cooking and a couple of other fire hazards

    A. True

    B. False

    C. Neither

31. The battery of the alarms needs to be charged at least _____ in a year

A. Twice

B. Checked

C. Once

32. Politeness and simplicity is the only manners needed in conducting proper phone etiquette

    A. True

    B. False

    C. Neither

33. With aging the risk for falling increases because their senses dim and nervous systems tends to deteriorate

    A. True

    B. False

    C. Neither

34. It is true that most of the falls lead to minor injuries, but at the same time nearly _____

to _____ percent lead to fractures as well as other serious injuries

A. Ten, sixty

B. Ten, fifty

C. Ten, seventy

35. Injuries that can result out of falls are broken bones, head injuries and even accidents that harm the interior body parts

A. True

B. False

C. Neither

36. _____ is a common form of dementia in which a person faces problem with their memory or thought process

A. Lupus

B. COPD

C. Alzheimer's

37. The symptoms of Alzheimer's are divided in two categories: _____ stage and _____ stage

    A. Late, noon

    B. Early, late

    C. Early, evening

38. The emotional support needs to come from the side of the caregiver and this can create a sense of wellbeing in the patient

    A. True

    B. False

    C. Neither

39. The early stage of Alzheimer attacks the patient so badly that they are not even in a position to communicate properly and they are completely dependent on the caregiver

    A. True

B. False

C. Neither

40. Memory loss in the Alzheimer's disease doesn't mean that the patient loses their feelings

A. True

B. False

C. Neither

41. The last stage of Alzheimer's completely cripples a person both mentally as well as physically

A. True

B. False

C. Neither

42. _____ is a brain disorder that deals with an abnormal self-absorption with oneself

A. Alzheimer's

B. Mad cow

C. Autism

43. Autistic children tend to play repetitive games with toys for example lining up of objects and the turning on and off of light switches despite repeated scolding

A. True

B. False

C. Neither

44. Some physical characteristic of autism may include

A. They are neat and well behave

B. They communicate with adults only

C. The skin is pale, face has low muscle tone

45. There is laboratory tests to confirm autism

A. True

B. False

C. Neither

46. The autistic patient may have fixations like making repeated noises, staring at turning wheels etc.

A. True

B. False

C. Neither

47. Autistic individuals often have good auditory processing skills

A. True

B. False

C. Neither

48. The high functioning autistic adults are very successful and they live relatively normal lives

A. True

B. False

C. Neither

49. The _____ adult autistics need constant care and attention like autistic children

A. Low functioning

B. High function

C. Normal functioning

Answers

1. A
2. B
3. C
4. B
5. B
6. C
7. A
8. B
9. A
10. B
11. A
12. A
13. B
14. C
15. C
16. A
17. B
18. C
19. B
20. A
21. C
22. B
23. B

24. A
25. C
26. B
27. C
28. B
29. A
30. B
31. A
32. C
33. B
34. A
35. B
36. A
37. C
38. B
39. A
40. B
41. A
42. A
43. C
44. A
45. C
46. B
47. A
48. B
49. A
50. A

ABOUT THE AUTHOR

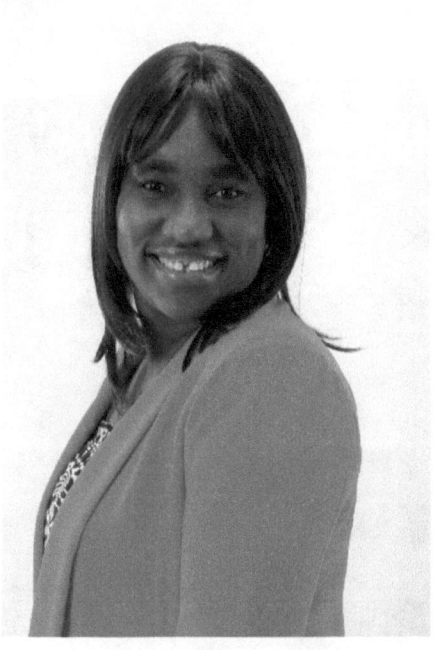

Jane John-Nwankwo is a Registered Nurse who loves to write. She has authored more than 20 books ranging from Textbooks to Exam Preparation materials, and now to fiction which is termed "Nurses' Romance Series"

Simply search
"Books by Jane John-Nwankwo"
On Amazon.com

Visit her website:
www.janejohn-nwankwo.com

Have you bought this book?

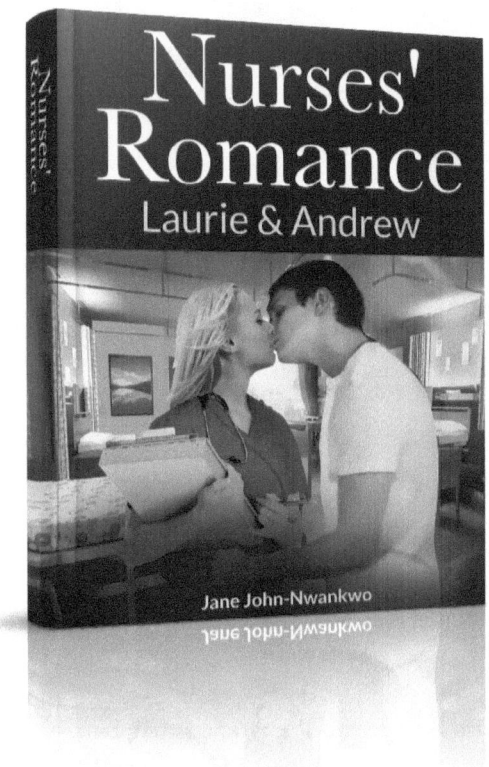

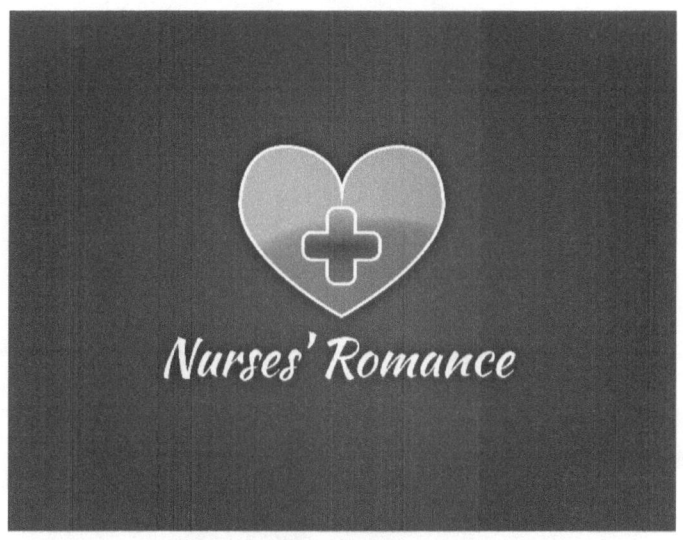

Visit www.janejohn-nwankwo.com

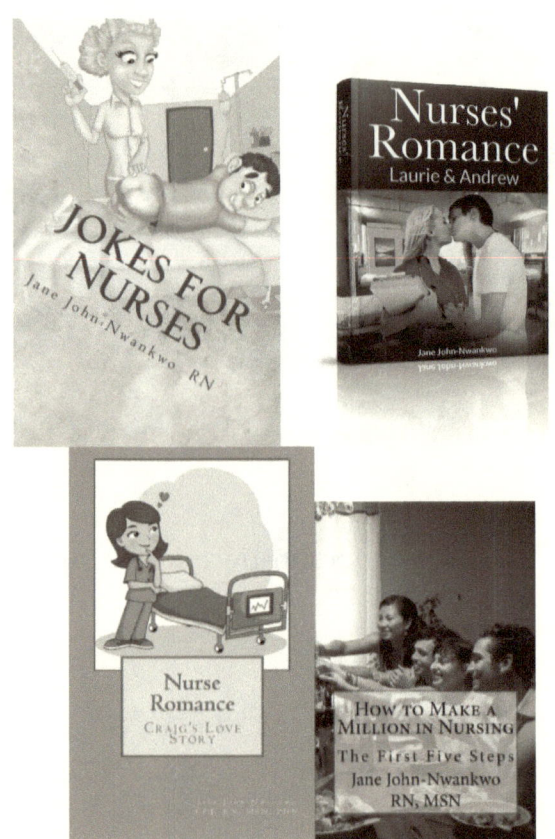

Have you purchased these books?

www.ingramcontent.com/pod-product-compliance
Lightning Source LLC
Chambersburg PA
CBHW032027290526
45786CB00011B/867